YOUR KNOWLEDGE HAS VALUE

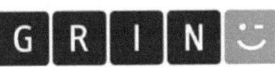

- We will publish your bachelor's and
  master's thesis, essays and papers

- Your own eBook and book -
  sold worldwide in all relevant shops

- Earn money with each sale

Upload your text at www.GRIN.com
and publish for free

GRIN ☺

Bibliographic information published by the German National Library:

The German National Library lists this publication in the National Bibliography; detailed bibliographic data are available on the Internet at http://dnb.dnb.de .

Imprint:

Copyright © 2011 GRIN Verlag, Open Publishing GmbH
Print and binding: Books on Demand GmbH, Norderstedt Germany
ISBN: 9783668474819

P. Ronald

Intensity Modulated Brachytherapy

GRIN Publishing

GRIN - Your knowledge has value

Since its foundation in 1998, GRIN has specialized in publishing academic texts by students, college teachers and other academics as e-book and printed book. The website www.grin.com is an ideal platform for presenting term papers, final papers, scientific essays, dissertations and specialist books.

Visit us on the internet:

http://www.grin.com/

http://www.facebook.com/grincom

http://www.twitter.com/grin_com

Contents

Intensity Modulated Brachytherapy

Radiotherapy

Radiation, the emission of rays of high frequency and wavelengths, has been in use for more than 100 years. It has been used in the field of medicine since the early 1900s when scientists like Marie Curie, who was awarded the Nobel Prize in Science for her cutting edge work in the field of radioactivity, discovered elements with radioactive properties such as radium and polonium. Since then, several new innovations have been made in the use of radiation in medicine. Radiation is majorly used in the treatment of cancers and malignant cells. And simply, radiotherapy can be defined as the use of ionizing radiation in the control and eradication of malignant cancer cells. It is to be differentiated from radiology which refers to the application of ionizing radiation in the diagnosis of diseases. Radiology makes use of radiation in the imaging of the human body.

There are two types of radiation, ionizing and non-ionizing radiation. Ionizing radiation has more applications in the field of radiotherapy than non-ionizing radiation. There are machines that can carefully measure doses of ionizing radiation and then direct the beams at the area of the body in which the cancerous cells are situated. These machines focus the high energy beams on the cells so as to either incapacitate them or totally destroy them. In most cases, these high energy beams damages certain parts of the cells, especially the DNA in the nucleus, thereby making these cells unable to divide and replicate. Unlike normal cells which can recover and repair themselves when damaged by radiation, cancerous cells cannot. And so they die.

The applications of radiotherapy are mainly in the treatment of cancer. However, the response of different forms of cancers to radiotherapy varies. The ability of a particular type of cancer to respond to radiation therapy is defined by its radiosensitivity which is the

2

intrinsic cellular sensitivity to ionizing radiation. Cancer cells with high radiosensitivities are quickly destroyed by minimal doses of radiation and types include the different types of germ cell tumours, leukaemia and lymphomas. Cancers with moderately radiosensitivities include almost all carcinomas (epithelial malignancies) while those with low radiosensitivities include melanomas and nephroblastomas. Also, the concept of "radiocurability", which is the likelihood of cure, alters a cancer's response to radiation. However, the two concepts are different in that radiocurability is a clinical parameter while radiosensitivity can be measured in the laboratory.

Just as much as radiation therapy has several advantages which include ability to destroy cancer cells without causing much harm to normal cells, ability to grant long-term benefits and prolong life; it has several disadvantages which could be early or late side effects. Some of the early side effects include destruction of epithelial lined surfaces (such as the skin, gastrointestinal mucosa, respiratory mucosa, ureters, etc), swelling and accumulation of fluid, and infertility (as a result of damage to the gonads). Late side effects include hair loss, tissue fibrosis, secondary malignancies, heart disease, and cognitive dysfunctions.

Radiotherapy can be conventionally divided into three major classes: external beam radiotherapy (EBRT) or teletherapy; sealed source therapy, also known as Brachytherapy; and unsealed or open source radiotherapy. The difference between these three divisions has to do with the position of the source of radiation. In external beam radiotherapy, the source of radiation is outside the body whereas in sealed source radiotherapy, the sources of radiation are sealed up and placed in the exact location of the area of the body to be irradiated. The sealed sources can either be injected, ingested orally or infused.

Brachytherapy

The word "brachytherapy" was derived from the Greek word 'brachy' which means 'within a short distance'. The concept of Brachytherapy has been referred to in different literatures as sealed source radiotherapy (as stated above), internal radiotherapy, curietherapy (from Madam Curie), or endocurie therapy. It "is a term used to describe the short distance treatment of cancer with radiation from small, encapsulated radionuclide sources" (Suntharalingam, Podgorsak, & Tölli, 2004). In this type of radiotherapy, the source of radiation is placed within or close to the area of interest which is to be irradiated. And in contrast to external beam radiotherapy in which high energy beams are focused on the cancerous part from outside the individual's body, brachytherapy requires precise placement of the sealed source directly at the location of the tumour. The radiation can then be delivered on and on for either a short period of time (using temporary implants) or for the lifetime of the sealed source till it decays (using permanent implants). Most of the radiation sources used in brachytherapy makes use of photons. However, in some situations, sources emitting beta rays or neutrons can be applied.

The use of brachytherapy can be dated back to the early 1900s when historical records revealed that Pierre Curie brought about the innovation of inserting a radioactive source into a cancerous tumour. And it was discovered that doing this made the tumour reduce in size. Also, Alexander Graham Bell made suggestions of treating cancers by direct implantation of sealed radioactive sources within cancerous tumours (Brenner 1997). Since then, several new innovations and modifications have been made to the use of brachytherapy to treat cancers.

Brachytherapy treatments can be classified in various ways. One of the ways of classification is based on the position of implants. And there are two main types: intracavitary and interstitial (Saito et al 2007). In intracavitary brachytherapy treatment, the source of

4

radiation is placed inside the body cavity closest to the cancerous tumour, unlike in the interstitial type in which the source is placed within the tumour itself. Another difference between these two is that intracavitary brachytherapy treatments are usually temporary whereas interstitial brachytherapy treatments have the ability to stay permanently, but may still be temporary. There are several other forms of brachytherapy treatments based on the type of implant, and these include surface (in which the source is placed on the tumour), intraoperative (in which the sources are placed within the target site during a surgical procedure), intravascular (in which the source, usually single, is placed within an artery either small or large), and intraluminal (in which the sources are placed within a lumen) (Suntharalingam, Podgorsak, & Tölli, 2004). Another mode of classification of brachytherapy treatments is based on the dose rate, and this has three classes: brachytherapy treatments with low dose rate (that is, between 0.4 – 2 Gy/h at the dose specification points), medium dose rate (2 – 12 Gy/h), and high dose rate (greater than 12 Gy/h) (Suntharalingam, Podgorsak, & Tölli, 2004). Based on the source loading, brachytherapy treatments can be divided into hot loading, in which the applicator of the radiation is preloaded and already contains radioisotopes at the time of insertion or implantation, and afterloading, in which the applicator is first implanted, then loaded later with the radioactive sources either manually or automatically (Suntharalingam, Podgorsak, & Tölli, 2004). A final method of classification is based on the duration of treatment – temporary and permanent implants. This classification has been discussed earlier.

Just like radiotherapy on its own, brachytherapy is mainly used in the treatment of cancers. Most commonly, brachytherapy is used to treat cervical, prostatic, breast and skin cancers. Nonetheless, it can be applied in the treatment of cancers of the brain, eye, gastrointestinal system, respiratory system, urinary and reproductive systems in both males and females (Saito et al 2007). Unlike external beam radiotherapy, sealed source radiotherapy allows the delivering of a high dose of radiation to a relatively smaller area. This is because of the ability to position sealed radiation sources precisely at the location of the tumour. Also, the sources or radiation maintain their position no matter the position of the individual receiving the treatment or of the tumour itself. This makes accurate targeting of the tumour possible and makes the physicians to achieve a very high level of radioactive dose conformity. Also, this ability causes a reduction in the risk of damage of healthy cells, tissues and organs which are in close proximity to the tumour, and thereby enhancing the possibility of cure and preservation of tissue, organ and systemic function.

Apart from the treatment of cancers, brachytherapy has also been applied in the treatment of coronary in-stent restenosis (Lee et al 1999). Usually, intravascular implants are used and are delivered via catheters. In addition, brachytherapy can be used in the treatment of other cardiovascular conditions such as atrial fibrillation and stenosis of peripheral vessels.

Just like radiotherapy, brachytherapy has its own advantages and disadvantages. Unlike radiotherapy, brachytherapy allows accurate distribution of radiation, especially to the tumour to be destroyed, and it also reduces the risk of irradiation of normal cells, tissues and organs. Also, instead of an individual coming for several episodes of irradiation with high energy beams, a permanent implant can be placed either within the tumour or close to the tumour as possible which delivers the necessary dose of radiation much more efficiently. Nonetheless, it has its own side effects which may be acute or late (long-term). Some of the acute side effects include uncontrolled bleeding, tissue swelling, bruising and pains or discomfort in the area of implantation (Saito et al 2007). There may also be feelings of fatigue and tiredness following implantation. Some of the long term side effects include erectile dysfunction, digestive system dysfunction, urinary problems, scar tissue formation, fat necrosis, etc.

Intensity Modulated Radiotherapy

The subject of radiation therapy has evolved over the years from older, archaic techniques to more sophisticated techniques. And it is a well known fact that using radiation to treat cancers is very tricky. The main aim of radiotherapy is to deliver as much dose of radiation as possible to a cancerous tissue in order to destroy it, and at the same time, trying to spare nearby non-malignant tissue which may be very radiosensitive. This has been a hard nut to crack for scientists for several years until the advent of intensity modulated radiotherapy.

Intensity modulated radiotherapy is a subset of external beam radiotherapy which makes use of high energy beams, especially X-rays, to destroy cancerous cells. In the earlier stages of the evolution of radiotherapy, conventional external beam radiotherapy was being used to deliver X-radiation via linear accelerators. The beams are usually being delivered through 2D (two-dimensional) beams with a single beam reaching the client from several directions. It may be from the back, front, or either side (laterally). This method is still in use in many centres as the conventional X-ray machines for taking chest, cranial, abdominal radiographs. However, the major drawback of this method is the delivery of high dose radiation which is needed to destroy cancerous tissue to normal healthy tissues which are in close proximity. For instance, irradiation of a prostatic carcinoma via this method exposes adjacent rectal tissue to the same dose of radiation. In order to combat this, the concept of three-dimensional conformal radiotherapy was being developed.

The three-dimensional conformal radiotherapy (designated 3DCRT) was a better replacement of the 2D conventional external beam radiotherapy. The concept of this version was to profile the shape of each beam of radiation to fit the exact profile of the target site. This focuses the beams of radiation exactly on the tumour site with a relative reduction in the amount of radiation delivered to surrounding tissues. This also provides the advantage of delivering higher doses of radiation to the cancerous tissue with less concerns of radiation toxicity to normal tissues in close proximity when compared to older conventional techniques. Nonetheless, despite the relatively safer nature of the 3D conformal radiotherapy, it cannot be compared to the high-precision nature of intensity modulated radiotherapy.

Intensity modulated radiotherapy is also a type of external beam radiation therapy in which the radiation beam is divided into several tiny rays that differ in intensity which pierce the body from multiple angles to intersect on the cancerous tissue. It further aids the ability to alter the treatment dose to both convex and concave tissue shapes. It also allows the delivery of a high dose of radiation to the cancerous tissue without damaging surrounding healthy tissue.

The main goal of intensity modulated radiotherapy is to cause dose escalation on the target and/or a dose reduction on nearby normal tissues (Hoveijn 2005). And it achieves this by assuming a greater control over the distribution of radiation dose in the client by intensity modulation. The intensity modulation in this method of radiotherapy is about inverse planning and optimization. All the clinician does is to outline the tumour site on a 3D simulation image, preferably a computed tomographic image. The planner, usually the radiologist, then enters the appropriate dose of radiation necessary to destroy the tumour as well as gives allowance for the surrounding healthy tissues. "Inverse treatment planning software using a computer optimized algorithm then arrives at the radiation beam characteristics most likely to meet the requirements designated at the start of treatment planning" (Lee & Terezakis 2008). Several other possibilities can be combined to see which would offer the optimum treatment plan that can give the best dose coverage while still reducing the dosage to healthy tissues at the lowest minimum.

There are several techniques which can be applied to achieve intensity modulated beams. One of these techniques is by using a multileaf collimator which in itself can be applied using two general methods. "The first is based on the sequential exposure of sub-beams or segments for which the collimators are (automatically) positioned while the radiation beam is switched off" (Williams 2003). This method is conventionally known as the multiple static field method, but has been referred to as the 'step and shoot' method. As each segment is being irradiated, the collimators are then moved on to the exact position for the following segment and then irradiated again. This process goes on and on until intensity modulation has been achieved. Unlike the first general method, the second method uses continuous irradiation. During the process of irradiation, each segment of the collimator moves based on a predefined trajectory at a specific point in time in order to achieve the desired intensity modulation. This method is being conventionally called the dynamic multileaf collimation method.

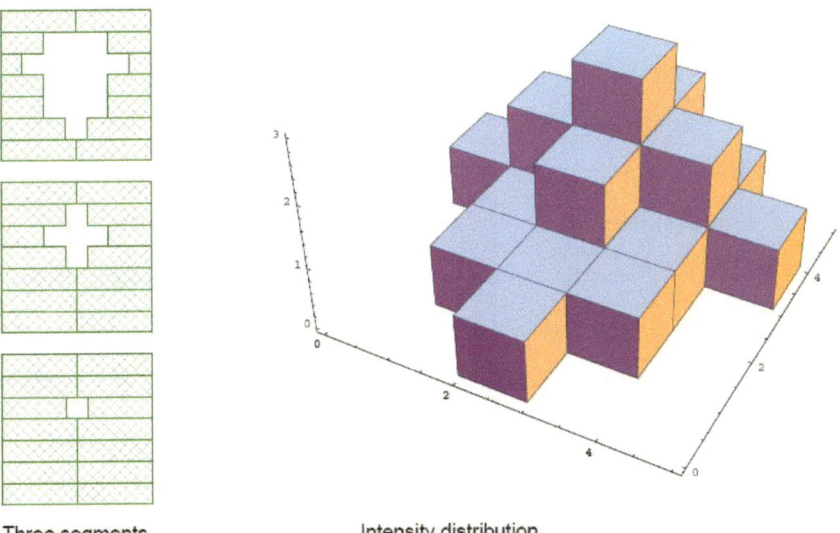

Three segments   Intensity distribution

Figure 1. Illustration of the multiple segment multileaf collimator. Source: Hoveijn 2005

The second technique is tomotherapy in which the "rotation of a series of fan beams around a patient generates a dose distribution within a slice, analogous to the slice thickness of a tomographic scanner" (Williams 2003). This technique applies the concept of three-dimensional imaging in a computerised tomographic scanner in which multiple image slices are taken in order to reconstruct them and generate a three-dimensional representation of the individual's body. So likewise, "in order to build up a three dimensional dose distribution in tomotherapy it is necessary to irradiate a series of slices between which the patient is moved by the slice width along the axis of rotation" (Williams 2003). Apart from this, there are other similarities between tomotherapy and computerised tomography. The axial resolution of the images taken via CT scanners is being limited by the thickness of each image slice taken, likewise in tomotherapy, the thickness of each image slice limits the axial resolution of the radiation dose distribution. This technique is being widely used, and it is being claimed that a significant proportion of intensity modulated radiotherapy treatments worldwide make use of the tomographic technique (although there are no recent data to back it up).

The planning of treatment with intensity modulated radiotherapy requires the coordinating clinician to delineate a sharp dose gradient around the predefined target volume. "As a result, the definition of appropriate volumes at risk for disease is of utmost importance to avoid a marginal miss without over-treating normal tissues" (Lee 2008). In order to achieve this, the physician and radiologists must make use of all available diagnostic tools at their disposal from the history and physical examination itself to the use of endoscopic and radiologic imaging studies (diagnostic computerised tomography scan, magnetic resonance imaging, and positron emission tomography scan). This is necessary to provide precise and adequate information about the tumour site and other possible regions of metastases. "Multidisciplinary discussion with a neuroradiologist, nuclear medicine physician, head and neck surgeon, and medical oncologist helps corroborate findings and aids in tumour volume delineation" (Lee 2008).

The use of intensity modulated radiotherapy has spread all over the world and a lot of studies conclude that it is a safe, successful and efficient form of therapy for different types of cancers. An investigation conducted by Gomez et al (2010) tried to compare the dose distribution in intensity modulated radiation therapy with conventional two-dimensional and three-dimensional conformal radiation therapy for early stage larynx cancers. From the three representative patients on whom multiple treatment plans were generated, the conclusion was that "IMRT provides a more ideal dose distribution compared to 2D treatment and 3D planning in regards to mean carotid dose" (Gomez et al, 2010). And therefore, it was recommended that intensity modulated radiotherapy should be used especially in situations where the physician is confident of the target volume.

In the treatment of head and neck cancers, intensity modulated radiation therapy has also demonstrated favourable outcomes. One of such is the conclusion made by Lee et al. who "published a series of 67 patients with nasopharyngeal carcinoma treated with IMRT and demonstrated a 4-year local progression-free and regional progression-free rate of 97% and 98% respectively" (Lee 2008). Also, another study carried out on 126 patients who presented with head and neck cancers, out of which 90% were either stage three or four, at Washington University, St. Louis by Chao et al. revealed that an 85% locoregional control rate was achieved after treatment with intensity modulated radiotherapy (Lee & Terezakis 2008).

Nonetheless, intensity modulated radiotherapy also has its own drawbacks. The efficiency of the therapy, as regards the tumour volume, is entirely dependent on the area predefined by the clinician. Unless a sharp dose gradient is selected, the risk of delivering

11

radiation to areas outside the predefined areas increases. Also, as is common with most advanced technologies, the financial cost of installing intensity modulated radiotherapy facilities is very high. It also requires a high level of expertise and a relatively longer staff delivery time.

Intensity modulated radiotherapy can be very effective in the management of malignancies as it cures more clients and harms less clients.

Intensity Modulated Brachytherapy

Intensity modulated brachytherapy is a treatment method which is very much similar to the concept behind intensity modulated radiotherapy. As stated earlier, brachytherapy requires the placement of the source of radiation within or close to the tumour as possible, in contrast to radiotherapy in which the source of the radiation is external to the body. Also, a major feature of brachytherapy is its ability to minimise radiation delivery to nearby surrounding tissues and focus directly on a localised area encircling the source of the radiation (Niehoff et al 2006). In addition, another advantage of brachytherapy over radiotherapy is its ability to stand steadfast and maintain its initial position relative to the tumour when there is movement of the client or the tumour itself during the course of treatment (Nohara et al 2010). All these show clearly the advantages of brachytherapy over conventional external beam radiotherapy. And its use has been successful in the treatment of various types of cancers. Unlike the other forms of treatment where a client has to keep coming for several visits to the treatment centre, those on brachytherapy need to make only a few visits and the procedure can even be performed in an outpatient setting. However, despite the several advantages of brachytherapy, it has its own clinical and technical challenges. And this has lead to the development of more efficient techniques, one of which is intensity modulated brachytherapy.

Some of the anatomic limitations of brachytherapy is that critical structures are sometimes close to the target site and the narrow physical space cannot allow the implantation or placement of larger equipment. Also, source limitations include the fact that the "radiation source will irradiate radiation in 4π geometry, source is hard to modulate, and the source will decay" (Shi 2011). These and other limitations have lead to the development of intensity modulated brachytherapy.

Intensity modulated brachytherapy was patterned after intensity modulated radiotherapy which was found to "improve dose uniformity within targets and to provide better sparing to the critical structures" (Cheng 2010). Due to the efficiency of intensity modulated radiotherapy, it has become a common practice in the field of radiotherapy. However, the use of intensity modulation in brachytherapy is still at the early stages with inadequate experimental studies.

Actually, the main aim of intensity modulated brachytherapy is to deliver a high dose of radiation to the target structure and at the same time minimise the dose delivered to adjacent healthy tissue. For instance, the smallest distance between the balloon and the ribs in Fig 1(a) was 0.4cm while that between the balloon and the skin was 1.1cm. And despite this close distance, radiation was not meant to be delivered to these tissues in close proximity. In order to achieve this, several approaches can be applied in the treatment planning to approximate and calculate the exact dose of radiation, and modulate the radiation delivery to avoid adjacent structures.

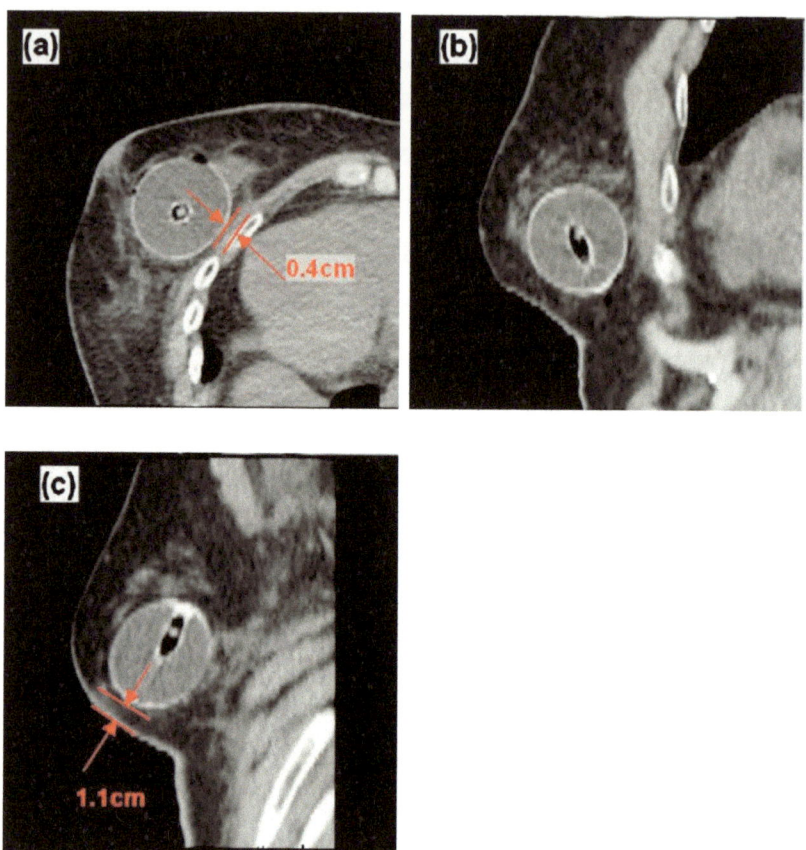

Figure 2. Computerised tomographic images showing (a) transverse, (b) coronal and (c) sagittal views of the chest wall. Source: Shi et al (2010)

One of the current approaches of intensity modulated brachytherapy is to use directional sources of radiation with partial blocks in order to produce a "fan beam" irradiation and create an irregularly shaped target as illustrated in Fig. 3 below (Shi, 2011). And it has been found out that "improved dose uniformity inside the target and better sparing to the adjacent normal structures can be achieved" (Shi et al 2010).

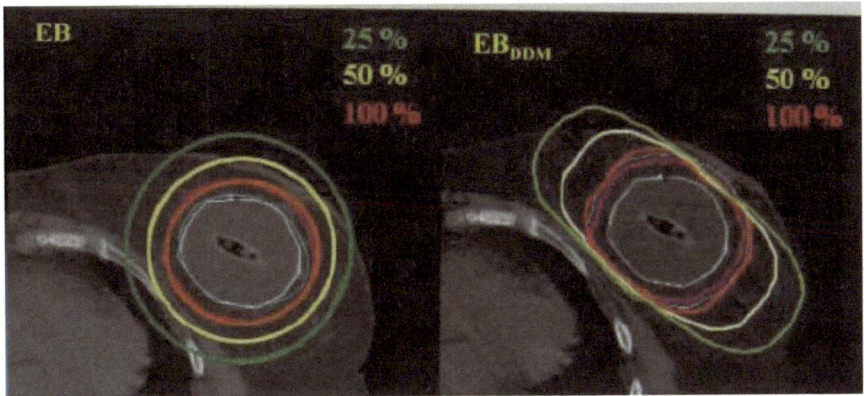

Figure 3. Illustration of the fan beam radiation produced by using directional sources with partial blocks.

One of the studies in this regard was performed by Ebert who made use of one dimensional intensity modulation in his conceptual study of brachytherapy treatment planning (Shi et al 2010). He used a partially shielded source which produced irradiation in fan beam geometry. Although there was a bit of scattering effect, it was disregarded. In this experiment, angular intensity modulation was achieved by performing an indexed rotation of the sealed source about its own axis. And from this, "a two dimensional (2D) and a three dimensional (3D) treatment plan were developed using a simulated annealing (SA) optimization algorithm and conformity based objective function" (Shi et al, 2010). Based on these results, Ebert's conclusion was that for tumour target sites which had irregular structures, a better dose conformity to the irregularly-shaped tumour can be achieved by angular intensity modulation.

In another study, "Lin et al. (2008, quoted in Shi et al 2010, p.3726) constructed a directional iodine-125 (I-125) source in a way that a gold shield was placed adjacent to the radioactive material within the encapsulation of the source" (Shi et al, 2010). And instead of a fan beam geometric irradiation which was produced by Ebert's experiment, the radiation emitted by the sealed source was nearly semispheral. By using Monte Carlo simulations, Lin et al was able to calculate the dose distribution surrounding the sealed source. In subsequent practical applications, the authors were able to achieve a lower dose in the surrounding tissues and a better dose uniformity inside the target itself. In an advancement of this method, Chaswal et al, using the same sealed source Lin et al made use of, "developed an optimization method for the planning using directional I-125 sources based on a greedy heuristic (GH) optimization algorithm and a region of interest adjoint objective function" (Shi et al, 2010). Their results showed a better sparing of the adjoining tissues, particularly the rectum and the urethra, with the use of directional sources in low dose rate prostate interstitial implants.

The above preliminary studies have shown that treatment plan quality can be improved with intensity modulation in brachytherapy. However, its use in actual clinical practice has been limited due to several factors. One of these factors is the rather limited space offered by the client's tissue for the insertion or implantation of the source (Niehoff et al 2006). In comparison to external beam radiotherapy, the radiation sources for brachytherapy are inserted either within tissues (interstitial) or placed inside body cavities (intracavitary). Apart from this, the use of intensity modulation in brachytherapy would inevitably prolong the treatment period. In intensity modulated radiotherapy, this challenge can be overcome by increasing the dose rate of the source, but this cannot be done in brachytherapy. Radioisotopes are usually made use of as sealed sources, and to increase the dose rate just as can be done in intensity modulated radiotherapy would mean increasing the specific activity which is impossible. Nonetheless, these limitations may be overcome with the advent of new advanced modifications.

The use of low energy sources with very high radiation output has thrown aside the limitations and has made clinical applications of intensity modulated brachytherapy possible. "Instead of radioactive isotopes, electronic brachytherapy sources use miniature X-ray tubes which offer adjustable x-ray energies" (Shi et al, 2010). A prototype has been developed by Xoft, particularly the Xoft Axxent™ X-ray source. It consists of a HV connector, HV cable, the source of the X-rays, the cooling sheath and a cooling inlet/outlet. The United States Food and Drug Administration (FDA) has approved the use of this model in accelerated partial breast irradiation. "Clinical studies have shown that compared to Ir-192 source, Xoft Axxent S700 source offers comparable coverage to the target and much lower dose to the normal tissues, though higher dose inhomogeneity in the target" (Shi et al, 2010). Also, another recent research using a heterogeneous virtualised human tumour revealed that Xoft, Inc's Axxent S700 source can minimise the doses to surrounding organs and tissues relative to using an Ir-192 source.

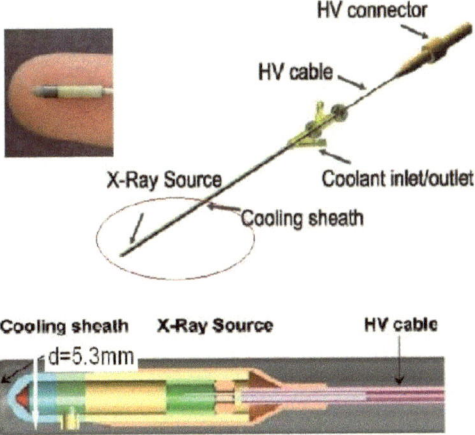

Figure 4. A schematic representation of Xoft's Axxent S700 X-ray source. Inset: actual size of the source.

While several studies have been carried out with intensity modulation in brachytherapy, there are still several limitations associated with this method. Most of the present applications of intensity modulated brachytherapy are restricted to using 1D angular intensity modulations. This means that the source's intensity can only be altered along a single direction, specifically along the azimuthal angle (using a spherical coordinate system) or the polar angle (using a collimator system) (Tepel et al 2005). In order to fully make use of the benefits of intensity modulated brachytherapy, a three-dimensional modulation offers more prospects. And if this is to be implemented, special planning methods involving the characterization of the source, dosimetry, and treatment planning are necessary.

The feasibility of three dimensional modulations in brachytherapy was investigated by Shi et al. The prototype treatment plan they designed consisted of "(1) A comprehensive source characterization method for IMBT based on Monte Carlo simulations; (2) a "modified TG-43" (mTG-43) dose calculation formalism developed specifically for IMBT dosimetry; (3) an inverse IMBT treatment planning method based on dose volume histogram (DVH) and dose surface histogram (DSH) constraints and a simulated annealing optimization algorithm" (Shi et al, 2010). The feasibility of intensity modulated brachytherapy was studied using ten patients with accelerated partial breast irradiation. The results of the study showed that intensity modulated brachytherapy improved the general plan quality for all the ten cases.

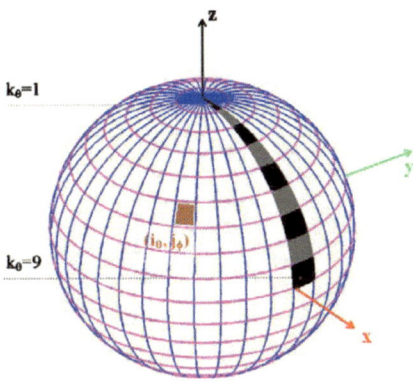

Figure 5. An illustration of the algorithm used for calibrating the intensity source. Source: Shi et al, 2010

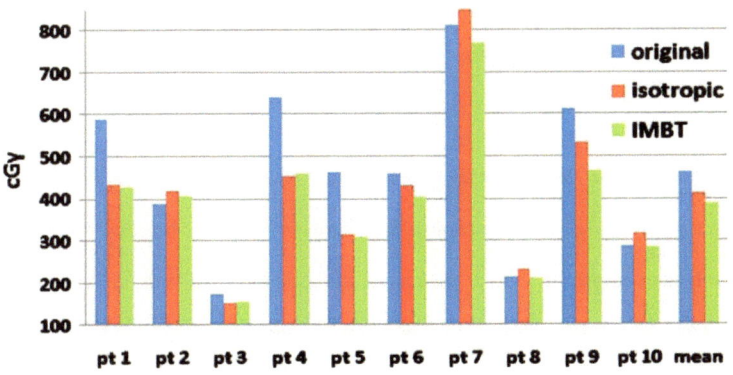

Figure 6. Graph showing the maximum dose delivered to the adjoining skin. Source: Shi et al 2010

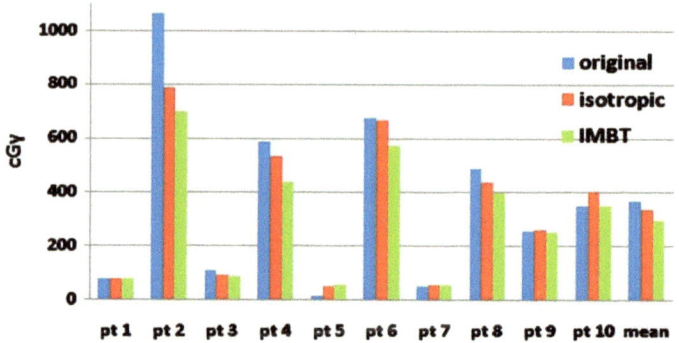

Figure 7. Graph showing the maximum dose delivered to the adjoining ribs. Source: Shi et al 2010

The graphs shown in Figs. 6 and 7 show a reduction in the maximum dose delivered to the skin and ribs with the use of intensity modulated brachytherapy when compared to the original and isotropic treatment plans.

All these studies have shown that there are a lot of benefits inherent in the clinical application of intensity modulated brachytherapy. But there are still some practical problems that need to be solved as regards the actual delivery of the technique to clients and that there is still a lot to learn. At present, there is no commercial collimator which can be used to produce single beamlets from the source. Also, there is also the challenge of prolonged treatment period. In addition, there is no quality assurance of the whole procedure itself (Tepel et al 2005). New innovations that would make a lot of difference in the application of intensity modulated brachytherapy would be machines with very high intensity modulation and high output sources which can efficiently deliver the required dose of radiation.

Conclusion

This review has been able to extensively discuss the trends in the field of radiotherapy from conventional external beam radiotherapy to innovations such as intensity modulated radiotherapy, and then focus on the nitty grity of intensity modulated brachytherapy. The use of radiation in the treatment of cancerous tissue is well known, but the risk of radiation toxicity to adjoining healthy tissues has given a lot of concern. This led to the development of more efficient radiation delivery sources which can deliver high doses of radiation to the target tissue, and at the same time minimise to the lowest possible level the amount of radiation delivered to healthy tissues.

Despite these new advances in the treatment of malignancies, these techniques have their own drawbacks which would need to be overcome before a very high quality assurance can be achieved. More investigations carried out in these fields would answer the questions that need to be answered and further refine the planning strategies, intraoperative techniques, and post-procedure evaluation in order to achieve a high level of treatment quality.

Bibliography

Brenner, D.J. (1997) Radiation Biology in Brachytherapy. Journal of Surgical Oncology, 65: pp.66–70.

Gomez, D. Cahlon, O. Mechalakos, J. & Lee, L. (2010) An investigation of intensity-modulated radiation therapy versus conventional two-dimensional and 3D-conformal radiation therapy for early stage larynx cancer. Radiation Oncology 2010, 5:74

Hoveijn, I. (2005) Intensity Modulated Radiation Therapy. Zeegse, June 2005: p.1/24

Lee, D.P. Lo, S. Forster, K. Yeung, A.C. & Oesterle, S.N. (1999) Clinical applications of brachytherapy for the prevention of restenosis. Vascular Medicine, 4: pp.257–268

Lee, N.Y. & Terezakis, S.A. (2008) Intensity-Modulated Radiation Therapy. Journal of Surgical Oncology 97: pp.691–696

Mehta, S.R. Suhag, V. Semwal, M. & Sharma, N. (2010) Radiotherapy: Basic Concepts and Recent Advances. MJAFI, 66: pp.158-162

Niehoff, P. Dietrich, J. Ostertag, H. Schmid, A. Kohr, P. Kimmig, B. Kovács, G. (2006) High-Dose-Rate (HDR) or Pulsed-Dose-Rate (PDR) Perioperative Interstitial Intensity-Modulated Brachytherapy (IMBT) for Local Recurrences of Previously Irradiated Breast or Thoracic Wall Following Breast Cancer. Strahlenther Onkol, 182: pp.102–7

Nohara, T. Mizokami, A. Kumano, T. Shigehara, K. Konaka, H. Yoshifumi, K. Yasuhide, K. Izumi, K. Narimoto, K & Namiki, M. (2010) Clinical Results of Iridium-192 High Dose Rate Brachytherapy with External Beam Radiotherapy. Japanese Journal of Clinical Oncology, doi:10.1093/jjco/hyq016

Saito, S. Nagata, H. Kosugi, M. Toya, K. Yorozu, A. Saito, S. Nagata, H. Kosugi, M. Toya, K. & Yorozu, A. (2007) Brachytherapy with permanent seed implantation. International Journal of Clinical Oncology, 12: pp.395–407

Shi, C. (2011) Three Dimensional Intensity Modulated Brachytherapy (IMBT): Dosimetry Algorithm and Inverse Treatment Planning. ppt

Shi, C. Guo, B. Cheng, C. Esquivel, C. Eng, T. & Papanikolaou. (2010) Three dimensional intensity modulated brachytherapy (IMBT): Dosimetry algorithm and inverse treatment planning. American Association of Physicists in Medicine, 37(7): pp.3725-3737

Suntharalingam, N. Podgorsak, E.B. & Tölli, H. Brachytherapy: Physical and Clinical Aspects

Tepel, J. Niehoff, P. Bokelmann, F. Faendrich, F. Kremer, B. Schmid, A. Kovács, G. (2005) Feasibility and Early Results of Interstitial Intensity-Modulated HDR/PDR Brachytherapy (IMBT) with/without Complementary External-Beam Radiotherapy and Extended Surgery in Recurrent Pelvic Colorectal Cancer. Strahlenther Onkol, 181: pp.696–703

Williams, P.C. (2003) IMRT: delivery techniques and quality assurance. The British Journal of Radiology, 76 (2003): pp.766–776

YOUR KNOWLEDGE HAS VALUE

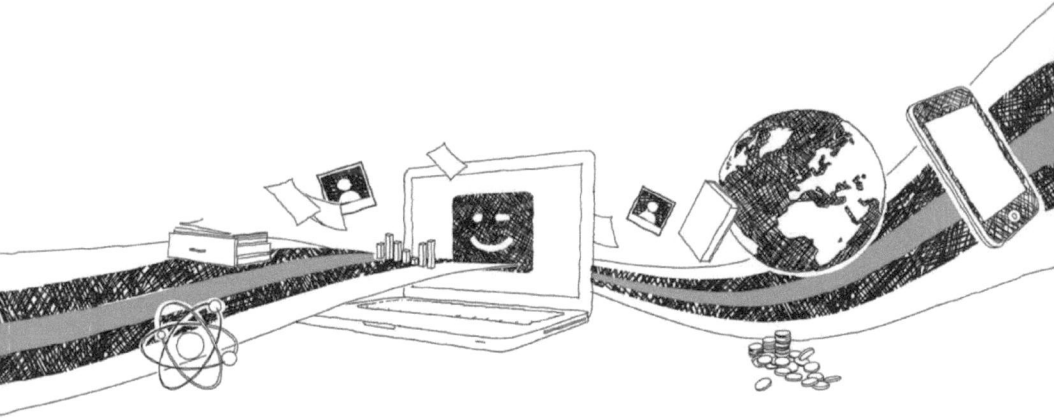

- We will publish your bachelor's and master's thesis, essays and papers

- Your own eBook and book - sold worldwide in all relevant shops

- Earn money with each sale

Upload your text at www.GRIN.com and publish for free

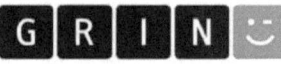